CONTENTS

INTRODUCTION

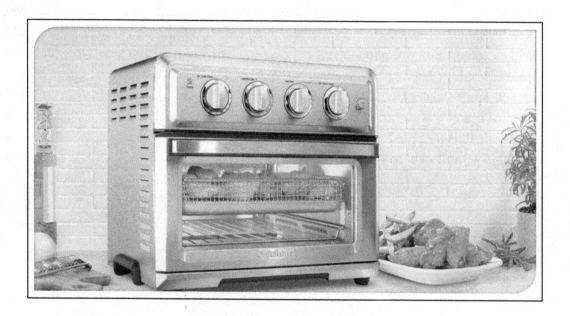

The Cuisinart AirFryer Toaster Oven is now available in a new, space-saving design! Cuisinart's Compact AirFryer Toaster Oven is big enough to airfry up to 2.5 lb. of food, toast 4 slices of bread or bagel halves, and bake up to a 3 lb. chicken. With all the features of our full-size models, including 6 functions and temperatures up to 450°F, this is an oven that offers multiple menu options and great performance without crowding the countertop!

Cuisinart AirFryer Toaster Oven, An even more miraculous ability is the air-frying function. Instead of cooking with oil, an air fryer uses really hot air to the same effect, yielding food that's just as crisp and golden but without the grease (though you can add a little oil for extra crunch). You can use it to make mini frozen pork dumplings oil-free, which came out crunchy and hot in less than ten minutes, or French- and sweet-potato fries, You could air-fry just about everything, like the kale to make homemade kale chips. The Cuisinart's toast function also works as well as, or better than, a stand-alone toaster, and its ovenlike design makes it easier to toast open-faced sandwiches or enough English muffins for three.

This unique kitchen workhorse is actually a premium full size toaster oven with a built-in airfryer. That means it not only bakes, broils, and toasts, it also lets you airfry right inside the oven. Air frying, which uses powerful ultra-hot air, is a healthier way to prepare delicious fried favorites, from wings to fritters to fries to shrimp. And since toaster ovens stay on the countertop, this fryer doesn't have to move back and forth, from cupboard to counter. Enjoy the crunch without the calories and messy cleanup, with the AirFryer Toaster Oven!

BREAKFAST AND BRUNCH RECIPES

SALTY PARSNIP PATTIES

Total Time: 20 minutes
Serves: 2

Ingredients

- 1 large parsnip, grated
- 3 eggs, beaten
- ½ tsp garlic powder
- ¼ tsp nutmeg
- 1 tbsp olive oil
- 1 cup flour
- Salt and black pepper to taste

Directions

In a bowl, combine flour, eggs, parsnip, nutmeg, and garlic powder. Season with salt and pepper. Form patties out of the mixture. Drizzle the AirFryer basket with olive oil and arrange the patties inside. Fit in the baking tray and cook for 15 minutes on Air Fry function at 360 F. Serve with garlic mayo.

GIANT STRAWBERRY PANCAKE

Total Time: 30 minutes

Serves: 3

Ingredients
- 3 eggs, beaten
- 2 tbsp butter, melted
- ½ cup flour
- 2 tbsp sugar, powdered
- ½ cup milk
- 1 ½ cups fresh strawberries, sliced

Directions
1. Preheat Cuisinart on Bake function to 350 F. In a bowl, mix flour, milk, eggs, and vanilla until fully incorporated. Add the mixture a greased with melted butter pan.
2. Place the pan in your toaster oven and cook for 12-16 minutes until the pancake is fluffy and golden brown. Drizzle powdered sugar and toss sliced strawberries on top.

QUICK PAPRIKA EGGS

Total Time: 10 minutes

Serves: 4

Ingredients

- 4 large eggs
- 1 tsp paprika
- Salt and pepper to taste
- ¼ cup cottage cheese, crumbled

Directions

Preheat your Cuisinart fryer to 350 F on Bake function. Crack an egg into a muffin cup. Repeat with the remaining cups. Sprinkle with salt and pepper. Top with cottage cheese. Put the cups in the Air Fryer tray and bake for 8-10 minutes. Remove and sprinkle with paprika to serve.

PARSLEY ONION & FETA TART

Total Time: 30 minutes
Serves: 4

Ingredients

- 3 ½ pounds Feta cheese
- Black pepper to taste
- 1 whole onion, chopped
- 2 tbsp parsley, chopped
- 1 egg yolk
- 5 sheets frozen filo pastry

Directions

1. Cut each of the 5 filo sheets into three equal-sized strips. Cover the strips with oil. In a bowl, mix onion, pepper, feta, salt, egg yolk, and parsley.
2. Make triangles using the cut strips and add a little bit of the feta mixture on top of each triangle. Place the triangles in a greased baking sheet and cook for 5 minutes at 400 F on Bake function. Serve sprinkled with green onions.

CLASSIC CHEDDAR CHEESE OMELET

Total Time: 15 minutes
Serves: 1

Ingredients

- 2 eggs, beaten
- Black pepper to taste
- 1 cup cheddar cheese, shredded
- 1 whole onion, chopped
- 2 tbsp soy sauce

Directions

1. Preheat Cuisinart on Air Fry function to 340 F. In a bowl, mix the eggs with soy sauce, salt, and pepper. Stir in the onion and cheddar cheese.
2. Pour the egg mixture in a greased baking pan and cook for 10-12 minutes. Serve and enjoy!

TOMATO, BASIL & MOZZARELLA BREAKFAST

Total Time: 10 minutes

Serves: 1

Ingredients

- 2 slices of bread
- 4 tomato slices
- 4 mozzarella slices
- 1 tbsp olive oil
- 1 tbsp chopped basil
- Salt and black pepper to taste

Directions

Preheat Cuisinart on Toast function to 350 F. Place the bread slices in the toaster oven and toast for 5 minutes. Arrange two tomato slices on each bread slice. Season with salt and pepper.

FRESH KALE & COTTAGE OMELET

Total Time: 15 minutes
Serves: 1

Ingredients

- 3 eggs
- 3 tbsp cottage cheese
- 3 tbsp chopped kale
- ½ tbsp chopped basil
- ½ tbsp chopped parsley
- Salt and black pepper to taste
- 1 tsp olive oil

Directions

Beat the eggs with salt and pepper in a bowl. Stir in the rest of the ingredients. Drizzle a baking pan with olive oil. Pour in the mixture and place it into the Cuisinart oven. Cook for 10-12 minutes on Bake function at 360 F until slightly golden and set. Serve.

BUTTERED APPLE & BRIE CHEESE SANDWICH

Total Time: 10 minutes

Serves: 1

Ingredients

- 2 bread slices
- ½ apple, thinly sliced
- 2 tsp butter
- 2 oz brie cheese, thinly sliced

Directions

Spread butter on the bread slices. Top with apple slices. Place brie slices on top of the apples. Finish with the other slice of bread. Cook in Cuisinart for 5 minutes at 350 F on Bake function.

HERBY PARMESAN BAGEL

Total Time: 10 minutes
Serves: 1

Ingredients

- 2 tbsp butter, softened
- 1 tsp dried basil
- 1 tsp dried parsley
- 1 tsp garlic powder
- 1 tbsp Parmesan cheese
- Salt and black pepper to taste
- 1 bagel

Directions

1. Preheat Cuisinart on Bake function to 370 degrees. Cut the bagel in half. Combine the butter, Parmesan cheese, garlic, basil, and parsley in a small bowl. Season with salt and pepper. Spread the mixture onto the bagel. Place the bagel in a baking pan and cook for 5 minutes. Serve.
2. Top each slice with 2 mozzarella slices. Return to the oven and cook for 1 minute more. Drizzle the caprese toasts with olive oil and top with chopped basil.

VANILLA & CINNAMON TOAST TOPPET

Total Time: 10 minutes
Serves: 6

Ingredients
- 12 slices bread
- ½ cup sugar
- 1 ½ tsp cinnamon
- 1 stick of butter, softened
- 1 tsp vanilla extract

Directions
Preheat Cuisinart on Toast function to 360 F. Combine all ingredients, except the bread, in a bowl. Spread the buttery cinnamon mixture onto the bread slices. Place the bread slices in the toaster oven. Cook for 8 minutes. Serve.

CINNAMON-ORANGE TOAST

Total Time: 15 minutes
Serves: 6

Ingredients

- 12 slices bread
- ½ cup sugar
- 1 stick butter
- 1½ tbsp vanilla extract
- 1½ tbsp cinnamon
- 2 oranges, zested

Directions

Mix butter, sugar, and vanilla extract and microwave for 30 seconds until everything melts. Add in orange zest. Pour the mixture over bread slices. Lay the bread slices in your Cuisinart Air Fryer pan and cook for 5 minutes at 400 F on Toast function. Serve with berry sauce.

PROSCIUTTO & MOZZARELLA CROSTINI

Total Time: 7 minutes
Serves: 1

Ingredients

- ½ cup finely chopped tomatoes
- 3 oz chopped mozzarella
- 3 prosciutto slices, chopped
- 1 tbsp olive oil
- 1 tsp dried basil
- 6 small slices of French bread

Directions

Preheat Cuisinart on Toast function to 350 F. Place the bread slices in the toaster oven and toast for 5 minutes. Top the bread with tomatoes, prosciutto and mozzarella. Sprinkle the basil over the mozzarella. Drizzle with olive oil. Return to oven and cook for 1 more minute, enough to become melty and warm.

PORRIDGE WITH HONEY & PEANUT BUTTER

Total Time: 15 minutes
Serves: 4

Ingredients

- 2 cups steel-cut oats
- 1 cup flax seeds
- 1 tbsp peanut butter
- 1 tbsp butter
- 4 cups milk
- 4 tbsp honey

Directions

Preheat Cuisinart on Bake function to 390 F. Combine all of the ingredients in an ovenproof bowl. Place in a baking pan and cook for 7 minutes. Stir and serve.

PEPPERY SAUSAGE & PARSLEY PATTIES

Total Time: 20 minutes
Serves: 4

Ingredients

- 1 lb ground Italian sausage
- ¼ cup breadcrumbs
- 1 tsp dried parsley
- 1 tsp red pepper flakes
- ½ tsp salt
- ¼ tsp black pepper
- ¼ tsp garlic powder
- 1 egg, beaten

Directions

Preheat Cuisinart on Bake function to 350 F. Combine all of the ingredients in a large bowl. Line a baking sheet with parchment paper. Make patties out of the sausage mixture and arrange them on the baking sheet. Cook for 15 minutes, flipping once halfway through cooking. Serve.

HONEY BANANA PASTRY WITH BERRIES

Total Time: 15 minutes
Serves: 2

Ingredients

- 3 bananas, sliced
- 3 tbsp honey
- 2 puff pastry sheets, cut into thin strips
- Fresh berries to serve

Directions

Preheat Cuisinart on Bake function to 340 F. Place the banana slices into a baking dish. Cover with the pastry strips and top with honey. Cook for 12 minutes. Serve with berries.

POULTRY RECIPES

SAVORY BUFFALO CHICKEN

Total Time: 35 minutes
Serves: 4

Ingredients
- 2 pounds chicken wings
- ½ cup cayenne pepper sauce
- ½ cup coconut oil
- 1 tbsp Worcestershire sauce
- 1 tbsp kosher salt

Directions

In a bowl, mix cayenne pepper sauce, coconut oil, Worcestershire sauce, and salt; set aside. Place chicken in the Air Fryer basket and fit in the baking tray. Cook for 25 minutes at 380 F on Air Fy function. Transfer to a large-sized plate and drizzle with the prepared sauce to serve.

GARLIC-BUTTERY CHICKEN WINGS

Total Time: 20 minutes
Serves: 4

Ingredients

- 12 chicken wings
- ¼ cup butter
- ¼ cup honey
- ½ tbsp salt
- 4 garlic cloves, minced
- ¾ cup potato starch

Directions

Preheat Cuisinart on Air Fry function to 370 F. Coat chicken with potato starch. Transfer to the greased Air Fryer basket and fit in the baking tray. Cook for 5 minutes. Whisk the rest of the ingredients in a bowl. Pour the sauce over the wings and serve.

ROSEMARY CHICKEN BREASTS

Total Time: 15minutes

Serves: 2

Ingredients

- 2 chicken breasts
- Salt and black pepper to taste
- ½ cup dried rosemary
- 1 tbsp butter, melted

Directions

1. Preheat Cuisinart on Air Fry function to 390 F. Lay a foil on a flat surface. Place the breasts on the foil, sprinkle with rosemary, tarragon, salt, and pepper and and drizzle the butter.

2. Wrap the foil around the breasts. Place the wrapped chicken in the AirFryer basket and fit in the baking tray; cook for 12 minutes. Remove and carefully unwrap. Serve with the sauce extract and steamed veggies.

ENCHILADA CHEESE CHICKEN

Total Time: 25 minutes
Serves: 3

Ingredients

- 3 cups chicken breasts, chopped
- 2 cups cheese, grated
- ½ cup salsa
- 1 can green chilies, chopped
- 12 flour tortillas
- 2 cans enchilada sauce

Directions

In a bowl, mix salsa and enchilada sauce. Toss in the chopped chicken to coat. Place the chicken on the tortillas and roll; top with cheese. Place the prepared tortillas in a baking tray and cook for 15-18 minutes at 400 F on Bake function. Serve with guacamole and hot dips!

BASIL MOZZARELLA CHICKEN

Total Time: 25 minutes

Serves: 4

Ingredients

- 4 chicken breasts, cubed
- 4 basil leaves
- ¼ cup balsamic vinegar
- 4 slices tomato
- 1 tbsp butter
- 4 slices mozzarella cheese

Directions

Heat butter and balsamic vinegar in a pan over medium heat. Pour over the chicken. Place the chicken in a baking pan and cook for 20 minutes at 400 F on Bake function. Top with cheese, and Bake for 1 minute until the cheese melts. Cover with basil and tomato slices and serve.

LIME-CHILI CHICKEN WINGS

Total Time: 25 minutes
Serves: 2

Ingredients

- 9 chicken wings
- 2 tbsp hot chili sauce
- ½ tbsp lime juice
- ½ tbsp honey
- ½ tbsp kosher salt
- ½ tbsp black pepper

Directions

Preheat Cuisinart on Air Fry function to 350 F. Mix the lime juice, honey, and chili sauce. Toss the mixture over the chicken wings. Put the chicken wings in the basket and fit in the baking tray; cook for 25 minutes. Shake every 5 minutes. Serve.

CHICKEN WITH AVOCADO & RADISH BOWL

Total Time: 20 minutes

Serves: 2

Ingredients

- 2 chicken breasts
- 1 avocado, sliced
- 4 radishes, sliced
- 1 tbsp chopped parsley
- Salt and black pepper to taste

Directions

Preheat Cuisinart on Air Fry function to 300 F. Cut the chicken into small cubes. Combine all ingredients in a bowl and transfer to the Air Fryer pan. Cook for 14 minutes, shaking once. Serve with cooked rice or fried red kidney beans.

DELICIOUS COCONUT CHICKEN CASSEROLE

Total Time: 20 minutes
Serves: 4

Ingredients

- 2 large eggs, beaten
- 2 tbsp garlic powder
- Salt and black pepper to taste
- ¾ cup breadcrumbs
- ¾ cup shredded coconut
- 1 pound chicken tenders

Directions

Preheat your Cuisinart on Air Fry function to 400 F. Spray a baking sheet with cooking spray. In a deep dish, whisk garlic powder, eggs, pepper, and salt. In another bowl, mix the breadcrumbs and coconut. Dip your chicken tenders in egg mixture, then in the coconut mix; shake off any excess. Place the prepared chicken tenders in the greased basket and fit in the baking tray; cook for 12-14 minutes until golden brown. Serve.

SAVORY CHICKEN WITH ONION

Total Time: 20 minutes

Serves: 4

Ingredients

- 4 chicken breasts, cubed
- 1 ½ cup onion soup mix
- 1 cup mushroom soup
- ½ cup heavy cream

Directions

Preheat your Cuisinart oven to 400 F on Bake function. Add mushrooms, onion mix, and heavy cream in a frying pan. Heat on low heat for 1 minute. Pour the warm mixture over chicken and allow to sit for 25 minutes. Place the marinated chicken in the basket and fit in the baking tray; cook for 15 minutes. Serve and enjoy!

BASIL CHEESE CHICKEN

Total Time: 20 minutes
Serves: 4

Ingredients

- 4 chicken breasts, cubed
- 1 tbsp garlic powder
- 1 cup mayonnaise
- ½ tsp pepper
- ½ cup soft cheese
- ½ tbsp salt
- Chopped basil for garnish

Directions

In a bowl, mix cheese, mayonnaise, garlic powder, and salt to form a marinade. Cover your chicken with the marinade. Place the marinated chicken in the basket and fit in the baking tray; cook for 15 minutes at 380 F on Air Fry function. Serve garnished with chopped fresh basil.

CAYENNE CHICKEN WITH COCONUT FLAKES

Total Time: 25 minutes
Serves: 4

Ingredients

- 3 chicken breasts, cubed
- 3 cups coconut flakes
- 3 whole eggs, beaten
- ½ cup cornstarch
- Salt and black pepper to taste
- 1 tbsp cayenne pepper

Directions

In a bowl, mix salt, cornstarch, cayenne and black peppers. In another bowl, mix beaten eggs with coconut flakes. Dip the chicken in pepper mix, then in the egg mix. Cover with foil and place in the basket. Fit in the baking tray and cook for 20 minutes at 350 F on Air Fry function.

HONEY CHICKEN WINGS

Total Time: 25 minutes
Serves: 4

Ingredients

- 8 chicken drumsticks
- 2 tbsp sesame oil
- 4 tbsp honey
- 3 tbsp light soy sauce
- 2 crushed garlic clove
- 1 small knob fresh ginger, grated
- 1 small bunch cilantro, chopped
- 2 tbsp sesame seeds, toasted

Directions

Add all ingredients in a bowl, except sesame and cilantro. Massage until drumsticks are well coated. Preheat Cuisinart to 400 F on Air Fry. Place the drumsticks in the basket and fit in the baking tray; cook for 15 minutes, flipping once. Sprinkle with sesame seeds and cilantro. Serve.

GINGER CHICKEN WINGS

Total Time: 25 minutes

Serves: 3

Ingredients

- 1 pound chicken wings
- 1 tbsp cilantro
- Salt and black pepper to taste
- 1 garlic clove, minced
- 1 tbsp yogurt
- 2 tbsp honey
- ½ tbsp vinegar
- ½ tbsp ginger, minced

Directions

Preheat Cuisinart on Air Fry to 360 F. Season wings with salt and pepper, place them in the basket and fit in the baking tray. Cook for 15 minutes, shaking once. In a bowl, mix the remaining ingredients. Top the chicken with sauce and cook for 5 more minutes. Serve.

PARMESAN CHICKEN CUTLETS

Total Time: 30 minutes
Serves: 4

Ingredients

- ¼ cup Parmesan cheese, grated
- 4 chicken cutlets
- ⅛ tbsp paprika
- 2 tbsp panko breadcrumbs
- ½ tbsp garlic powder
- 2 large eggs, beaten

Directions

In a bowl, mix Parmesan cheese, breadcrumbs, garlic powder, and paprika. Add eggs to another bowl. Dip the chicken in eggs, dredge them in cheese mixture and place them in the basket and fit in the baking tray. Cook for 20-25 minutes on Air Fry function at 400 F.

BUTTERED CRISPY TURKEY

Total Time: 25 minutes
Serves: 4

Ingredients

- 1 pound turkey breast, halved
- 2 cups panko breadcrumbs
- Salt and black pepper to taste
- ½ tsp cayenne pepper
- 1 stick butter, melted

Directions

In a bowl, combine the breadcrumbs, salt, cayenne and black peppers. Brush the butter onto the turkey breast and coat in the crumb mixture. Transfer to a lined baking dish. Cook in your Cuisinart for 15 minutes at 390 F. Serve warm.

VEGETABLES RECIPES

GARLICKY BRUSSELS SPROUT

Total Time: 27 minutes

Serves: 4

Ingredients
- 1 lb. Brussels sprouts, cut in half
- 2 tablespoons oil
- 2 garlic cloves, minced
- ¼ teaspoon red pepper flakes, crushed
- Salt and ground black pepper, as required

Directions
1. In a bowl, add all the ingredients and toss to coat well.
2. Press "Power Button" of Air Fry Oven and turn the dial to select the "Air Fry" mode.
3. Press the Time button and again turn the dial to set the cooking time to 12 minutes.
4. Now push the Temp button and rotate the dial to set the temperature at 390 degrees F.
5. Press "Start/Pause" button to start.
6. When the unit beeps to show that it is preheated, open the lid.
7. Arrange the Brussels sprouts in "Air Fry Basket" and insert in the oven.
8. Serve hot.

SWEET & SOUR BRUSSELS SPROUT

Total Time: 20 minutes
Serves: 2

Ingredients

- 2 cups Brussels sprouts, trimmed and halved lengthwise
- 1 tablespoon balsamic vinegar
- 1 tablespoon maple syrup
- ¼ teaspoon red pepper flakes, crushed
- Salt, as required

Directions

1. In a bowl, add all the ingredients and toss to coat well.
2. Press "Power Button" of Air Fry Oven and turn the dial to select the "Air Fry" mode.
3. Press the Time button and again turn the dial to set the cooking time to 10 minutes.
4. Now push the Temp button and rotate the dial to set the temperature at 400 degrees F.
5. Press "Start/Pause" button to start.
6. When the unit beeps to show that it is preheated, open the lid.
7. Arrange the Brussels sprouts in "Air Fry Basket" and insert in the oven.
8. Serve hot.

SPICED EGGPLANT

Total Time: 40 minutes
Serves: 3

Ingredients

- 2 medium eggplants, cubed
- 2 tablespoons butter, melted
- 1 tablespoon Maggi seasoning sauce
- 1 teaspoon sumac
- 1 teaspoon garlic powder
- 1 teaspoon onion powder
- Salt and ground black pepper, as required
- 1 tablespoon fresh lemon juice
- 2 tablespoons Parmesan cheese, shredded

Directions

1. In a bowl, mix together the eggplant cubes, butter, seasoning sauce and spices. Press "Power Button" of Air Fry Oven and turn the dial to select the "Air Fry" mode.
2. Press the Time button and again turn the dial to set the cooking time to 15 minutes.
3. Now push the Temp button and rotate the dial to set the temperature at 320 degrees F. Press "Start/Pause" button to start.
4. When the unit beeps to show that it is preheated, open the lid.
5. Arrange the eggplant cubes in "Air Fry Basket" and insert in the oven.
6. After 15 minutes of cooking, toss the eggplant cubes.
7. Now, set the temperature at 320 degrees F for 10 minutes.
8. Transfer the eggplant cubes into a bowl with the lemon juice, and Parmesan and toss to coat well. Serve immediately.

HERBED EGGPLANT

Total Time: 30 minutes
Serves: 2

Ingredients

- ½ teaspoon dried marjoram, crushed
- ½ teaspoon dried oregano, crushed
- ½ teaspoon dried thyme, crushed
- ½ teaspoon garlic powder
- Salt and ground black pepper, as required
- 1 large eggplant, cubed
- Olive oil cooking spray

Directions

1. In a small bowl, mix together the herbs, garlic powder, salt, and black pepper.
2. Spray the eggplant cubes evenly cooking spray with and then, rub with the herbs mixture.
3. Press "Power Button" of Air Fry Oven and turn the dial to select the "Air Fry" mode.
4. Press the Time button and again turn the dial to set the cooking time to 15 minutes.
5. Now push the Temp button and rotate the dial to set the temperature at 390 degrees F.
6. Press "Start/Pause" button to start.
7. When the unit beeps to show that it is preheated, open the lid.
8. Arrange the eggplant cubes in "Air Fry Basket" and insert in the oven.
9. Spray the eggplant cubes with cooking spray 2 times.
10. Serve hot.

CURRIED EGGPLANT

Total Time: 30 minutes
Serves: 2

Ingredients

- 1 large eggplant, cut into ½-inch thick slices
- 1 garlic clove, minced
- ½ fresh red chili, chopped
- 1 tablespoon vegetable oil
- ¼ teaspoon curry powder
- Salt, as required

Directions

1. In a bowl, add all the ingredients and toss to coat well.
2. Press "Power Button" of Air Fry Oven and turn the dial to select the "Air Fry" mode.
3. Press the Time button and again turn the dial to set the cooking time to 15 minutes.
4. Now push the Temp button and rotate the dial to set the temperature at 300 degrees F.
5. Press "Start/Pause" button to start.
6. When the unit beeps to show that it is preheated, open the lid.
7. Arrange the eggplant cubes in "Air Fry Basket" and insert in the oven.
8. Serve hot.

HERBED POTATOES

Total Time: 26 minutes

Serves: 4

Ingredients

- 6 small potatoes, chopped
- 3 tablespoons olive oil
- 2 teaspoons mixed dried herbs
- Salt and ground black pepper, as required
- 2 tablespoons fresh parsley, chopped

Directions

1. In a large bowl, add the potatoes, oil, herbs, salt and black pepper and toss to coat well.
2. Press "Power Button" of Air Fry Oven and turn the dial to select the "Air Fry" mode.
3. Press the Time button and again turn the dial to set the cooking time to 16 minutes.
4. Now push the Temp button and rotate the dial to set the temperature at 355 degrees F.
5. Press "Start/Pause" button to start.
6. When the unit beeps to show that it is preheated, open the lid.
7. Arrange the potato pieces in "Air Fry Basket" and insert in the oven.
8. Garnish with parsley and serve.

JACKET POTATOES

Total Time: 30 minutes
Serves: 2

Ingredients

- 2 potatoes
- 1 tablespoon mozzarella cheese, shredded
- 3 tablespoons sour cream
- 1 tablespoon butter, softened
- 1 teaspoon chives, minced
- Salt and ground black pepper, as required

Directions

1. With a fork, prick the potatoes.
2. Press "Power Button" of Air Fry Oven and turn the dial to select the "Air Fry" mode.
3. Press the Time button and again turn the dial to set the cooking time to 15 minutes.
4. Now push the Temp button and rotate the dial to set the temperature at 355 degrees F.
5. Press "Start/Pause" button to start.
6. When the unit beeps to show that it is preheated, open the lid.
7. Arrange the potatoes in greased "Air Fry Basket" and insert in the oven.
8. Meanwhile, in a bowl, add the remaining ingredients and mix until well combined.
9. Transfer the potatoes onto a platter.
10. Open potatoes from the center and stuff them with cheese mixture.
11. Serve immediately

STUFFED POTATOES

Total Time: 46 minutes

Serves: 4

Ingredients

- 4 potatoes, peeled
- 2-3 tablespoons canola oil
- 1 tablespoon butter
- ½ of brown onion, chopped
- 2 tablespoons chives, chopped
- ½ cup Parmesan cheese, grated

Directions

1. Coat the potatoes with some oil. Press "Power Button" of Air Fry Oven and turn the dial to select the "Air Fry" mode. Press the Time button and again turn the dial to set the cooking time to 26 minutes.
2. Now push the Temp button and rotate the dial to set the temperature at 390 degrees F. Press "Start/Pause" button to start.
3. When the unit beeps to show that it is preheated, open the lid.
4. Arrange the potatoes in greased "Air Fry Basket" and insert in the oven.
5. Coat the potatoes twice with the remaining oil.
6. Meanwhile, in a frying pan, melt the butter over medium heat and sauté the onion for about 4-5 minutes.
7. Remove from the heat and transfer the onion into a bowl. In the bowl of onion, add the potato flesh, chives, and half of cheese and stir to combine.
8. After 20 minutes of cooking, press "Start/Pause" button to pause the unit and transfer the potatoes onto a platter.
9. Carefully, cut each potato in half. With a small scooper, scoop out the flesh from each half. Stuff the potato halves evenly with potato mixture and sprinkle with the remaining cheese. Arrange the potato halves in greased "Air Fry Basket" and insert in the oven. Serve immediately.

HASSELBACK POTATOES

Total Time: 50 minutes
Serves: 4

Ingredients

- 4 potatoes
- 2 tablespoons olive oil
- 2 tablespoons Parmesan cheese, shredded
- 1 tablespoon fresh chives, chopped

Directions

1. With a sharp knife, cut slits along each potato the short way about ¼-inch apart, making sure slices should stay connected at the bottom.
2. Gently brush each potato evenly with oil
3. Press "Power Button" of Air Fry Oven and turn the dial to select the "Air Fry" mode.
4. Press the Time button and again turn the dial to set the cooking time to 30 minutes.
5. Now push the Temp button and rotate the dial to set the temperature at 355 degrees F.
6. Press "Start/Pause" button to start.
7. When the unit beeps to show that it is preheated, open the lid.
8. Arrange the potatoes in greased "Air Fry Basket" and insert in the oven.
9. Coat the potatoes with the oil once halfway through.

10. Transfer the potatoes onto a platter and top with the cheeses, and chives.
11. Serve immediately.

POTATO GRATIN

Total Time: 35 minutes

Serves: 4

Ingredients

- 2 large potatoes, sliced thinly
- 5½ tablespoons cream
- 2 eggs
- 1 tablespoon plain flour
- ½ cup cheddar cheese, grated

Directions

1. Press "Power Button" of Air Fry Oven and turn the dial to select the "Air Fry" mode. Press the Time button and again turn the dial to set the cooking time to 10 minutes.
2. Now push the Temp button and rotate the dial to set the temperature at 355 degrees F. Press "Start/Pause" button to start.
3. When the unit beeps to show that it is preheated, open the lid.
4. Arrange the potato slices in "Air Fry Basket" and insert in the oven.
5. Meanwhile, in a bowl, add cream, eggs and flour and mix until a thick sauce forms. Remove the potato slices from the basket.
6. Divide the potato slices in 4 ramekins evenly and top with the egg mixture evenly, followed by the cheese.
7. Press "Power Button" of Air Fry Oven and turn the dial to select the "Air Fry" mode. Press the Time button and again turn the dial to set the cooking time to 10 minutes.
8. Now push the Temp button and rotate the dial to set the temperature at 390 degrees F.
9. Arrange the ramekins in "Air Fry Basket" and insert in the oven.
10. Press "Start/Pause" button to start. Serve warm.

STUFFED OKRA

Total Time: 27 minutes
Serves: 2

Ingredients

- 8 oz. large okra
- ¼ cup chickpea flour
- ¼ of onion, chopped
- 2 tablespoons coconut, grated freshly
- 1 teaspoon garam masala powder
- ½ teaspoon ground turmeric
- ½ teaspoon red chili powder
- ½ teaspoon ground cumin
- Salt, to taste

Directions

1. With a knife, make a slit in each okra vertically without cutting in 2 halves.
2. In a bowl, mix together the flour, onion, grated coconut, and spices.
3. Stuff each okra with the mixture.
4. Press "Power Button" of Air Fry Oven and turn the dial to select the "Air Fry" mode.
5. Press the Time button and again turn the dial to set the cooking time to 12 minutes.
6. Now push the Temp button and rotate the dial to set the temperature at 390 degrees F.
7. Press "Start/Pause" button to start.
8. When the unit beeps to show that it is preheated, open the lid.
9. Arrange the stuffed okra in "Air Fry Basket" and insert in the oven.
10. Serve hot.

STUFFED BELL PEPPERS

Total Time: 30 minutes

Serves: 5

Ingredients
- ½ small bell pepper, seeded and chopped
- 1 (15-oz.) can diced tomatoes with juice
- 1 (15-oz.) can red kidney beans, rinsed and drained
- 1 cup cooked rice
- 1½ teaspoons Italian seasoning
- 5 large bell peppers, tops removed and seeded
- ½ cup mozzarella cheese, shredded
- 1 tablespoon Parmesan cheese, grated

Directions
1. In a bowl, mix together the chopped bell pepper, tomatoes with juice, beans, rice, and Italian seasoning.
2. Stuff each bell pepper with the rice mixture.
3. Press "Power Button" of Air Fry Oven and turn the dial to select the "Air Fry" mode.
4. Press the Time button and again turn the dial to set the cooking time to 15 minutes.
5. Now push the Temp button and rotate the dial to set the temperature at 360 degrees F.
6. Press "Start/Pause" button to start.
7. When the unit beeps to show that it is preheated, open the lid.
8. Arrange the bell peppers in "Air Fry Basket" and insert in the oven.
9. Meanwhile, in a bowl, mix together the mozzarella and Parmesan cheese.
10. After 12 minutes of cooking, top each bell pepper with cheese mixture.
11. Serve warm.

STUFFED PUMPKIN

Total Time: 50 minutes
Serves: 5

Ingredients

- 1 sweet potato, peeled and chopped
- 1 parsnip, peeled and chopped
- 1 carrot, peeled and chopped
- ½ cup fresh peas, shelled
- 1 onion, chopped
- 2 garlic cloves, minced
- 1 egg, beaten
- 2 teaspoons mixed dried herbs
- Salt and ground black pepper, as required
- ½ of butternut pumpkin, seeded

Directions

1. In a large bowl, mix together the vegetables, garlic, egg, herbs, salt, and black pepper.
2. Stuff the pumpkin half with vegetable mixture.
3. Press "Power Button" of Air Fry Oven and turn the dial to select the "Air Fry" mode. Press the Time button and again turn the dial to set the cooking time to 30 minutes.
4. Now push the Temp button and rotate the dial to set the temperature at 355 degrees F.
5. Press "Start/Pause" button to start.
6. When the unit beeps to show that it is preheated, open the lid.
7. Arrange the pumpkin half in "Air Fry Basket" and insert in the oven.
8. Transfer the pumpkin onto a serving platter and set aside to cool slightly before serving.

VEGGIE RATATOUILLE

Total Time: 30 minutes

Serves: 4

Ingredients

- 1 green bell pepper, seeded and chopped
- 1 yellow bell pepper, seeded and chopped
- 1 eggplant, chopped
- 1 zucchini, chopped
- 3 tomatoes, chopped
- 2 small onions, chopped
- 2 garlic cloves, minced
- 2 tablespoons Herbs de Provence
- 1 tablespoon olive oil
- 1 tablespoon balsamic vinegar
- Salt and ground black pepper, as required

Directions

1. In a large bowl, add the vegetables, garlic, Herbs de Provence, oil, vinegar, salt, and black pepper and toss to coat well.
2. Transfer vegetable mixture into a greased baking pan.
3. Press "Power Button" of Air Fry Oven and turn the dial to select the "Air Fry" mode.
4. Press the Time button and again turn the dial to set the cooking time to 15 minutes.
5. Now push the Temp button and rotate the dial to set the temperature at 355 degrees F.
6. Press "Start/Pause" button to start.
7. When the unit beeps to show that it is preheated, open the lid.
8. Arrange the pan over the "Wire Rack" and insert in the oven.   Serve hot.

FISH AND SEAFOOD RECIPES

ROSEMARY BUTTERED PRAWNS

Total Time: 15 minutes
Serves: 2

Ingredients

- 8 large prawns
- 1 rosemary sprig, chopped
- ½ tbsp melted butter
- Salt and black pepper to taste

Directions

1. Combine butter, rosemary, salt, and pepper in a bowl. Add in the prawns and mix to coat. Cover the bowl and refrigerate for 1 hour.
2. Preheat Cuisinart on Air Fry function to 350 F Remove the prawns from the fridge and place them in the basket. Fit in the baking tray and cook for 10 minutes, flipping once. Serve.

PARMESAN FISH WITH PINE NUTS

Total Time: 15 minutes
Serves: 4

Ingredients
- 2 tbsp fresh basil, chopped
- 2 garlic cloves, minced
- 2 tbsp olive oil
- 1 tbsp Parmesan cheese, grated
- salt and black pepper to taste
- 2 tbsp pine nuts
- 4 white fish fillets
- 2 tbsp olive oil

Directions

Preheat Cuisinart on Air Fry function to 350 F. Season the fish with salt and pepper. Place in the greased basket and fit in the baking tray. Cook the fillets for 8 minutes, flipping once. In a bowl, add basil, olive oil, pine nuts, garlic, and Parmesan cheese; mix well. Serve with the fish.

DELIGHTFUL CATFISH FILLETS

Total Time: 25 minutes
Serves: 4

Ingredients
- 4 catfish fillets
- ¼ cup seasoned fish fry
- 1 tbsp olive oil
- 1 tbsp parsley, chopped

Directions
Add seasoned fish fry and catfish fillets in a large Ziploc bag and massage well to coat. Place the fillets in your Cuisinart Air Fryer basket and fit in the baking tray; cook for 10 minutes at 360 F on Air Fry function. Flip the fish and cook for 2-3 more minutes. Top with parsley and serve.

SHRIMP WITH SMOKED PAPRIKA & CAYENNE PEPPER

Total Time: 10 minutes

Serves: 3

Ingredients
- 6 oz tiger shrimp, 12 to 16 pieces
- 1 tbsp olive oil
- ½ a tbsp old bay seasoning
- ¼ a tbsp cayenne pepper
- ¼ a tbsp smoked paprika
- A pinch of sea salt

Directions
Preheat Cuisinart on Air Fry function to 380 F. Mix olive oil, old bay seasoning, cayenne pepper, smoked paprika, and sea salt in a large bowl. Add in the shrimp and toss to coat. Place the shrimp in the frying basket and fit in the baking tray; cook for 6-7 minutes, sahing once. Serve.

SPEEDY FRIED SCALLOPS

Total Time: 5 minutes
Serves: 4

Ingredients

- 12 fresh scallops
- 3 tbsp flour
- Salt and black pepper to taste
- 1 egg, lightly beaten
- 1 cup breadcrumbs

Directions

Coat the scallops with flour. Dip into the egg, then into the breadcrumbs. Spray with olive oil and arrange them on the basket. Fit in the baking tray and cook for 6 minutes at 360 F on Air Fry function, turning once halfway through cooking. Serve.

FRIED COD NUGGETS

Total Time: 25 minutes
Serves: 4

Ingredients

- 1 ¼ lb cod fillets, cut into 4 to 6 chunks each
- ½ cup flour
- 1 egg
- 1 cup cornflakes
- 1 tbsp olive oil
- Salt and black pepper to taste

Directions

Place the olive oil and cornflakes in a food processor and process until crumbed. Season the fish chunks with salt and pepper. In a bowl, beat the egg along with 1 tbsp of water. Dredge the chunks in flour first, then dip in the egg, and finally coat with cornflakes. Arrange the fish pieces on a lined sheet and cook in your Cuisinart on Air Fry at 350 F for 15 minutes until crispy.

SAVORY COD FISH IN SOY SAUCE

Total Time: 20 minutes
Serves: 4

Ingredients

- 4 cod fish fillets
- 4 tbsp chopped cilantro
- Salt to taste
- 2 green onions, chopped
- 1 cup water
- 4 slices of ginger
- 4 tbsp light soy sauce
- 3 tbsp oil
- 1 tsp dark soy sauce
- 4 cubes rock sugar

Directions

1. Sprinkle the cod with salt and cilantro and drizzle with olive oil. Place in the cooking basket and fit in the baking tray; cook for 15 minutes at 360 F on Air Fry function.
2. Place the remaining ingredients in a frying pan over medium heat and cook for 5 minutes until sauce reaches desired consistency. Pour the sauce over the fish and serve.

CRISPY CRAB LEGS

Total Time: 15 minutes
Serves: 4

Ingredients
- 3 pounds crab legs
- ½ cup butter, melted

Directions
Preheat Cuisinart on Air Fry function to 380 F. Cover the crab legs with salted water and let them stay for a few minutes. Drain, pat them dry, and place the legs in the basket. Fit in the baking tray and brush with some butter; cook for 10 minutes, flipping once. Drizzle with the remaining butter and serve.

QUICK SHRIMP BOWL

Total Time: 15 minutes
Serves: 4

Ingredients
- 1 ¼ pounds tiger shrimp
- ¼ tsp cayenne pepper
- ½ tsp old bay seasoning
- ¼ tsp smoked paprika
- A pinch of salt
- 1 tbsp olive oil

Directions
Preheat your Cuisinart oven to 390 F on Air Fry function. In a bowl, mix all the ingredients. Place the mixture in your the cooking basket and fit in the baking tray; cook for 5 minutes, flipping once. Serve drizzled with lemon juice.

GARLIC-BUTTER CATFISH

Total Time: 20 minutes
Serves: 2

Ingredients
- 2 catfish fillets
- 2 tsp blackening seasoning
- Juice of 1 lime
- 2 tbsp butter, melted
- 1 garlic clove, mashed
- 2 tbsp cilantro

Directions
In a bowl, blend in garlic, lime juice, cilantro, and butter. Pour half of the mixture over the fillets and sprinkle with blackening seasoning. Place the fillets in the basket and fit in the baking tray; cook for 15 minutes at 360 F on Air Fry function. Serve the fish with remaining sauce.

DELICIOUS FRIED SEAFOOD

Total Time: 15 minutes

Serves: 4

Ingredients

- 1 lb fresh scallops, mussels, fish fillets, prawns, shrimp
- 2 eggs, lightly beaten
- Salt and black pepper to taste
- 1 cup breadcrumbs mixed with zest of 1 lemon

Directions

1. Dip each piece of the seafood into the eggs and season with salt and pepper. Coat in the crumbs and spray with oil. Arrange into the frying basket and fit in the baking tray; cook for 10 minutes at 400 F on Air Fry function, turning once halfway through. Serve.

EASY SALMON CAKES

Total Time: 15 minutes
Serves: 2

Ingredients
- 8 oz salmon, cooked
- 1 ½ oz potatoes, mashed
- A handful of capers
- A handful of parsley, chopped
- Zest of 1 lemon
- 1 ¾ oz plain flour

Directions
1. Carefully flake the salmon in a bowl. Stir in zest, capers, dill, and mashed potatoes. Shape the mixture into cakes and dust them with flour. Place in the fridge for 60 minutes.
2. Preheat your Cuisinart to 350 F on Air Fry function. Remove the cakes from the fridges and arrange them on the greased basket. Fit in the baking tray and cook for 10 minutes, shaing once halfway through. Serve chilled.

OLD BAY TILAPIA FILLETS

Total Time: 15 minutes

Serves: 4

Ingredients

- 1 pound tilapia fillets
- 1 tbsp old bay seasoning
- 2 tbsp canola oil
- 2 tbsp lemon pepper
- Salt to taste
- 2-3 butter buds

Directions

Preheat your Cuisinart oven to 400 F on Bake function. Drizzle tilapia fillets with canola oil. In a bowl, mix salt, lemon pepper, butter buds, and seasoning; spread on the fish. Place the fillet on the basket and fit in the baking tray. Cook for 10 minutes, flipping once until tender and crispy.

SWEET CAJUN SALMON

Total Time: 10 minutes
Serves: 1

Ingredients

- 1 salmon fillet
- ¼ tsp brown sugar
- Juice of ½ lemon
- 1 tbsp cajun seasoning
- 2 lemon wedges
- 1 tbsp chopped parsley

Directions

Preheat Cuisinart on Bake function to 350 F. Combine sugar and lemon juice; coat the salmon with this mixture. Coat with the Cajun seasoning as well. Place a parchment paper on a baking tray and cook the fish in your Cuisinart for 10 minutes. Serve with lemon wedges and parsley.

LEMON-GARLIC BUTTER LOBSTER

Total Time: 15 minutes
Serves: 2

Ingredients
- 4 oz lobster tails
- 1 tsp garlic, minced
- 1 tbsp butter
- Salt and black pepper to taste
- ½ tbsp lemon Juice

Directions
1. Add all the ingredients to a food processor except for lobster and blend well. Wash lobster and halve using a meat knife; clean the skin of the lobster and cover with the marinade.
2. Preheat your Cuisinart to 380 F on Air Fry function. Place the lobster in the cooking basket and fit in the baking tray; cook for 10 minutes. Serve with fresh herbs.

BANG BANG BREADED SHRIMP

Total Time: 24 minutes
Serves: 4

Ingredients

- 1 lb. raw shrimp peeled and deveined
- 1 egg white
- 1/2 cup flour
- 3/4 cup panko bread crumbs
- 1 teaspoon paprika
- Montreal Seasoning to taste
- salt and pepper to taste
- cooking spray

Bang Bang Sauce

- 1/3 cup Greek yogurt
- 2 tablespoon Sriracha
- 1/4 cup sweet chili sauce

Directions

1. Mix flour with salt, black pepper, paprika, and Montreal seasoning in a bowl.
2. Dredge the shrimp the flour then dip in the egg.
3. Coat the shrimp with the breadcrumbs and place them in an Air fryer basket.
4. Press "Power Button" of Air Fry Oven and turn the dial to select the "Air Roast" mode.
5. Press the Time button and again turn the dial to set the cooking time to 14 minutes. Now push the Temp button and rotate the dial to set the temperature at 400 degrees F.
6. Once preheated, place the Air fryer basket in the oven and close its lid.
7. Toss and flip the shrimp when cooked halfway through. Serve warm.

TACO FRIED SHRIMP

Total Time: 15 minutes
Serves: 6

Ingredients

- 17 shrimp, defrosted, peeled, and deveined
- 1 cup bread crumbs Italian
- 1 tablespoon taco seasoning
- 1 tablespoon garlic salt
- 4 tablespoon butter melted
- olive oil spray

Directions

1. Toss the shrimp with oil and all other ingredients in a bowl.
2. Spread the seasoned shrimp in the Air fryer Basket.
3. Press "Power Button" of Air Fry Oven and turn the dial to select the "Air Roast" mode.
4. Press the Time button and again turn the dial to set the cooking time to 5 minutes.
5. Now push the Temp button and rotate the dial to set the temperature at 400 degrees F.
6. Once preheated, place the Air fryer basket in the oven and close its lid.
7. Toss and flip the shrimp when cooked halfway through.
8. Serve warm.

GARLIC MUSSELS

Total Time: 16 minutes

Serves: 4

Ingredients

- 1 lb. mussels
- 1 tablespoon butter
- 1 cup of water
- 2 teaspoons minced garlic
- 1 teaspoon chives
- 1 teaspoon basil
- 1 teaspoon parsley

Directions

1. Toss the mussels with oil and all other ingredients in a bowl.
2. Spread the seasoned shrimp in the oven baking tray.
3. Press "Power Button" of Air Fry Oven and turn the dial to select the "Air Roast" mode.
4. Press the Time button and again turn the dial to set the cooking time to 6 minutes.
5. Now push the Temp button and rotate the dial to set the temperature at 390 degrees F.
6. Once preheated, place the mussel's tray in the oven and close its lid.
7. Serve warm.

MUSSELS WITH SAFFRON SAUCE

Total Time: 18 minutes

Serves: 4

Ingredients

- 1 tablespoon unsalted butter
- 1 tablespoon minced garlic
- 1 tablespoon minced shallot
- 1/4 cup dry white wine
- 3 tablespoons heavy cream
- 4 threads saffron
- 1 lb. fresh mussels

Directions

1. Whisk cream with saffron, shallots, white wine, and butter in a bowl.
2. Place the mussels in the oven baking tray and pour the cream sauce on top.
3. Press "Power Button" of Air Fry Oven and turn the dial to select the "Bake" mode.
4. Press the Time button and again turn the dial to set the cooking time to 8 minutes.
5. Now push the Temp button and rotate the dial to set the temperature at 370 degrees F.
6. Once preheated, place the mussel's baking tray in the oven and close its lid.
7. Serve warm.

CAJUN SHRIMP BAKE

Total Time: 50 minutes
Serves: 8

Ingredients

- 4 andouille sausages, chopped
- 1 lb. shrimp, peeled and deveined
- 4 red potatoes, quartered
- 2 pieces corn, quartered
- 2 tablespoons oil, divided
- 1 tablespoon butter, cubed
- 4 cloves garlic, minced

Cajun Spice Mix

- 2 teaspoons garlic powder
- 2 ½ teaspoons paprika
- 1 ¼ teaspoons dried oregano
- 1 teaspoon onion powder
- 1 ¼ teaspoons dried thyme
- ½ teaspoon red pepper flakes
- 1 teaspoon cayenne pepper
- 2 teaspoons salt
- 1 teaspoon pepper

Directions

1. Mix Cajun mix spices in a bowl and then toss in all the veggies and seafood.
2. Stir in sausage, corn, oil, and butter then mix well.
3. Spread potatoes, corn, and garlic in the oven baking tray.
4. Press "Power Button" of Air Fry Oven and turn the dial to select the "Bake" mode. Press the Time button and again turn the dial to set the cooking time to 25 minutes. Now push the Temp button and rotate the dial to set the temperature at 375 degrees F.
5. Once preheated, place the potato's baking tray in the oven and close its lid.
6. When potatoes are done, add shrimp and sausage to the potatoes.
7. Return the baking tray to the oven and bake for 15 minutes. Serve warm.

SHRIMP WITH GARLIC SAUCE

Total Time: 23 minutes

Serves: 4

Ingredients

- 1 1/4 lbs. shrimp, peeled and deveined
- 1/4 cup butter
- 1 tablespoon minced garlic
- 2 tablespoon fresh lemon juice
- Salt and pepper
- 1/8 teaspoon Red pepper flakes
- 2 tablespoon minced fresh parsley

Directions

1. Toss the shrimp with oil and all other ingredients in a bowl.
2. Spread the seasoned shrimp in the baking pan.
3. Press "Power Button" of Air Fry Oven and turn the dial to select the "Bake" mode.
4. Press the Time button and again turn the dial to set the cooking time to 13 minutes.
5. Now push the Temp button and rotate the dial to set the temperature at 350 degrees F.
6. Once preheated, place the baking pan in the oven and close its lid.
7. Serve warm.

SHRIMP SCAMPI

Total Time: 23 minutes
Serves: 8

Ingredients

- 2 lbs. jumbo shrimp, deveined and peeled
- 3 tablespoons olive oil
- 4 tablespoons lemon juice
- 2 teaspoons salt
- 1/2 teaspoon black pepper
- 1/4 cup butter
- 4 cloves garlic, minced
- 1 small shallot, minced
- 2 tablespoons minced fresh parsley
- 1/2 teaspoon dried oregano
- 1/4 teaspoon crushed red pepper flakes
- 1 egg yolk
- 2/3 cup panko bread crumbs

Directions

1. Toss shrimp with egg, spices, seasonings, oil, herbs, butter, and shallots in a bowl. Mix well, then add breadcrumbs to coat well.
2. Spread the shrimp in a baking tray in a single layer.
3. Press "Power Button" of Air Fry Oven and turn the dial to select the "Bake" mode. Press the Time button and again turn the dial to set the cooking time to 13 minutes.
4. Now push the Temp button and rotate the dial to set the temperature at 425 degrees F.
5. Once preheated, place the shrimp's baking tray in the oven and close its lid.
6. Toss and flip the shrimp when cooked halfway through.
7. Serve warm.

SHRIMP PARMESAN BAKE

Total Time: 18 minutes

Serves: 4

Ingredients

- 1 1/2 lb. large raw shrimp, peeled and deveined
- 1/4 cup melted butter
- 1 teaspoon coarse salt
- 1/4 teaspoon black pepper
- 1 teaspoon garlic powder
- 1/2 teaspoon crushed red pepper
- 1/4 cup Parmesan cheese, grated

Directions

1. Toss the shrimp with oil and all other ingredients in a bowl.
2. Spread the seasoned shrimp in the Baking tray.
3. Press "Power Button" of Air Fry Oven and turn the dial to select the "Bake" mode.
4. Press the Time button and again turn the dial to set the cooking time to 8 minutes.
5. Now push the Temp button and rotate the dial to set the temperature at 400 degrees F.
6. Once preheated, place the lobster's baking tray in the oven and close its lid.
7. Switch the Air fryer oven to broil mode and cook for 1 minute.
8. Serve warm.

BEEF,LAMB & PORK

BEEF SKEWERS WITH POTATO SALAD

Total Time: 35 minutes
Serves: 4

Ingredients
- juice ½ lemon
- 2 tablespoon olive oil
- 1 garlic clove, crushed
- 1 ¼ lb. diced beef

For the salad

- 2 potatoes, boiled, peeled and diced
- 4 large tomatoes, chopped
- 1 cucumber, chopped
- 1 handful black olives, chopped
- 9 oz. pack feta cheese, crumbled
- 1 bunch of mint, chopped

Directions
1. Whisk lemon juice with garlic and olive oil in a bowl.
2. Toss in beef cubes and mix well to coat. Marinate for 30 minutes.
3. Alternatively, thread the beef on the skewers.
4. Place these beef skewers in the Air fry basket. Press "Power Button" of Air Fry Oven and turn the dial to select the "Air fryer" mode.
5. Press the Time button and again turn the dial to set the cooking time to 25 minutes. Now push the Temp button and rotate the dial to set the temperature at 360 degrees F.
6. Once preheated, place the Air fryer basket in the oven and close its lid.
7. Flip the skewers when cooked halfway through then resume cooking.
8. Meanwhile, whisk all the salad ingredients in a salad bowl.
9. Serve the skewers with prepared salad.

CLASSIC SOUVLAKI KEBOBS

Total Time: 30 minutes
Serves: 6

Ingredients

- 2 ¼ lbs. beef shoulder fat trimmed, cut into chunks
- 1/3 cup olive oil
- ½ cup red wine
- 2 teaspoon dried oregano
- ½ cup of orange juice
- 1 teaspoon orange zest
- 2 garlic cloves, crushed

Directions

1. Whisk olive oil, red wine, oregano, oranges juice, zest, and garlic in a suitable bowl.
2. Toss in beef cubes and mix well to coat. Marinate for 30 minutes.
3. Alternatively, thread the beef, onion, and bread on the skewers.
4. Place these beef skewers in the Air fry basket.
5. Press "Power Button" of Air Fry Oven and turn the dial to select the "Air fryer" mode.
6. Press the Time button and again turn the dial to set the cooking time to 20 minutes.
7. Now push the Temp button and rotate the dial to set the temperature at 370 degrees F.
8. Once preheated, place the Air fryer basket in the oven and close its lid.
9. Flip the skewers when cooked halfway through then resume cooking.
10. Serve warm.

HARISSA DIPPED BEEF SKEWERS

Total Time: 26 minutes
Serves: 6

Ingredients

- 1 lb. beef mince
- 4 tablespoon harissa
- 2 oz. feta cheese
- 1 large red onion, shredded
- 1 handful parsley, chopped
- 1 handful mint, chopped
- 1 tablespoon olive oil
- juice 1 lemon

Directions

1. Whisk beef mince with harissa, onion, feta, and seasoning in a bowl.
2. Make 12 sausages out of this mixture then thread them on the skewers.
3. Place these beef skewers in the Air fry basket.
4. Press "Power Button" of Air Fry Oven and turn the dial to select the "Bake" mode.
5. Press the Time button and again turn the dial to set the cooking time to 16 minutes.
6. Now push the Temp button and rotate the dial to set the temperature at 370 degrees F.
7. Once preheated, place the Air fryer basket in the oven and close its lid.
8. Flip the skewers when cooked halfway through then resume cooking.
9. Toss the remaining salad ingredients in a salad bowl.
10. Serve beef skewers with tomato salad.

ONION PEPPER BEEF KEBOBS

Total Time: 30 minutes

Serves: 4

Ingredients

- 2 tablespoon pesto paste
- 2/3 lb. beefsteak, diced
- 2 red peppers, cut into chunks
- 2 red onions, cut into wedges
- 1 tablespoon olive oil

Directions

1. Toss in beef cubes with harissa and oil, then mix well to coat. Marinate for 30 minutes.
2. Alternatively, thread the beef, onion, and peppers on the skewers.
3. Place these beef skewers in the Air fry basket.
4. Press "Power Button" of Air Fry Oven and turn the dial to select the "Air fryer" mode.
5. Press the Time button and again turn the dial to set the cooking time to 20 minutes.
6. Now push the Temp button and rotate the dial to set the temperature at 370 degrees F.
7. Once preheated, place the Air fryer basket in the oven and close its lid.
8. Flip the skewers when cooked halfway through then resume cooking.
9. Serve warm.

MAYO SPICED KEBOBS

Total Time: 20 minutes

Serves: 4

Ingredients

- 2 tablespoon cumin seed
- 2 tablespoon coriander seed
- 2 tablespoon fennel seed
- 1 tablespoon paprika
- 2 tablespoon garlic mayonnaise
- 4 garlic cloves, finely minced
- ½ teaspoon ground cinnamon
- 1 ½ lb. lean minced beef

Directions

1. Blend all the spices and seeds with garlic, cream, and cinnamon in a blender.
2. Add this cream paste to the minced beef then mix well.
3. Make 8 sausages and thread each on the skewers.
4. Place these beef skewers in the Air fry basket.
5. Press "Power Button" of Air Fry Oven and turn the dial to select the "Air fryer" mode.
6. Press the Time button and again turn the dial to set the cooking time to 10 minutes.
7. Now push the Temp button and rotate the dial to set the temperature at 370 degrees F.
8. Once preheated, place the Air fryer basket in the oven and close its lid.
9. Flip the skewers when cooked halfway through then resume cooking.
10. Serve warm.

BEEF WITH ORZO SALAD

Total Time: 37 minutes
Serves: 4

Ingredients

- 2/3 lbs. beef shoulder, cubed
- 1 teaspoon ground cumin
- ½ teaspoon cayenne pepper
- 1 teaspoon sweet smoked paprika
- 1 tablespoon olive oil
- 24 cherry tomatoes

Salad:

- ½ cup orzo, boiled
- ½ cup frozen pea
- 1 large carrot, grated
- small pack coriander, chopped
- small pack mint, chopped
- juice 1 lemon
- 2 tablespoon olive oil

Directions

1. Toss tomatoes and beef with oil, paprika, pepper, and cumin in a bowl.
2. Alternatively, thread the beef and tomatoes on the skewers.
3. Place these beef skewers in the Air fry basket. Press "Power Button" of Air Fry Oven and turn the dial to select the "Air fryer" mode.
4. Press the Time button and again turn the dial to set the cooking time to 25 minutes. Now push the Temp button and rotate the dial to set the temperature at 370 degrees F.
5. Once preheated, place the Air fryer basket in the oven and close its lid.
6. Flip the skewers when cooked halfway through then resume cooking.
7. Meanwhile, sauté carrots and peas with olive oil in a pan for 2 minutes.
8. Stir in mint, lemon juice, coriander, and cooked couscous.
9. Serve skewers with the couscous salad.

BEEF ZUCCHINI SHASHLIKS

Total Time: 35 minutes

Serves: 4

Ingredients

- 1lb. beef, boned and diced
- 1 lime, juiced and chopped
- 3 tablespoon olive oil
- 20 garlic cloves, chopped
- 1 handful rosemary, chopped
- 3 green peppers, cubed
- 2 zucchinis, cubed
- 2 red onions, cut into wedges

Directions

1. Toss the beef with the rest of the skewer's ingredients in a bowl.
2. Thread the beef, peppers, zucchini, and onion on the skewers.
3. Place these beef skewers in the Air fry basket.
4. Press "Power Button" of Air Fry Oven and turn the dial to select the "Air fryer" mode.
5. Press the Time button and again turn the dial to set the cooking time to 25 minutes.
6. Now push the Temp button and rotate the dial to set the temperature at 370 degrees F.
7. Once preheated, place the Air fryer basket in the oven and close its lid.
8. Flip the skewers when cooked halfway through then resume cooking.
9. Serve warm.

SPICED BEEF SKEWERS

Total Time: 28 minutes

Serves: 4

Ingredients

- 2 teaspoons ground cumin
- 2 teaspoons ground coriander
- 1/4 teaspoon ground cinnamon
- 1/8 teaspoon ground smoked paprika
- 2 teaspoons lime zest
- 1/2 teaspoon salt
- 1/2 teaspoon black pepper
- 1 tablespoon lemon juice
- 2 teaspoons olive oil
- 1 1/2 lbs. lean beef, cubed

Directions

1. Toss beef with the rest of the skewer's ingredients in a bowl.
2. Thread the beef and veggies on the skewers alternately.
3. Place these beef skewers in the Air fry basket.
4. Press "Power Button" of Air Fry Oven and turn the dial to select the "Air fryer" mode.
5. Press the Time button and again turn the dial to set the cooking time to 18 minutes.
6. Now push the Temp button and rotate the dial to set the temperature at 370 degrees F.
7. Once preheated, place the Air fryer basket in the oven and close its lid.
8. Flip the skewers when cooked halfway through then resume cooking.
9. Serve warm.

BEEF SAUSAGE WITH CUCUMBER SAUCE

Total Time: 25 minutes
Serves: 6

Ingredients

Beef Kabobs

- 1 lb. ground beef
- 1/2 an onion, finely diced
- 3 garlic cloves, finely minced
- 2 teaspoons cumin
- 2 teaspoons coriander
- 1 ½ teaspoons salt
- 2 tablespoons chopped mint

Yogurt Sauce:

- 1 cup Greek yogurt
- 2 tablespoons cucumber, chopped
- 2 garlic cloves, minced
- 1/4 teaspoon salt

Directions

1. Toss beef with the rest of the kebob ingredients in a bowl.
2. Make 6 sausages out of this mince and thread them on the skewers.
3. Place these beef skewers in the Air fry basket.
4. Press "Power Button" of Air Fry Oven and turn the dial to select the "Air fryer" mode. Press the Time button and again turn the dial to set the cooking time to 15 minutes. Now push the Temp button and rotate the dial to set the temperature at 370 degrees F.
5. Once preheated, place the Air fryer basket in the oven and close its lid.
6. Flip the skewers when cooked halfway through then resume cooking.
7. Meanwhile, prepare the cucumber sauce by whisking all its ingredients in a bowl. Serve the skewers with cucumber sauce.

BEEF EGGPLANT MEDLEY

Total Time: 30 minutes

Serves: 4

Ingredients

- 2 cloves of garlic
- 1 teaspoon dried oregano
- olive oil
- 4 beef steaks, diced
- 2 eggplant, cubed
- 8 fresh bay leaves
- 2 lemons, juiced
- a few sprigs parsley, chopped

Directions

1. Toss beef with the rest of the skewer's ingredients in a bowl.
2. Thread the beef and veggies on the skewers alternately.
3. Place these beef skewers in the Air fry basket.
4. Press "Power Button" of Air Fry Oven and turn the dial to select the "Air fryer" mode.
5. Press the Time button and again turn the dial to set the cooking time to 20 minutes.
6. Now push the Temp button and rotate the dial to set the temperature at 370 degrees F.
7. Once preheated, place the Air fryer basket in the oven and close its lid.
8. Flip the skewers when cooked halfway through then resume cooking.
9. Serve warm.

GLAZED BEEF KEBOBS

Total Time: 30 minutes
Serves: 6

Ingredients

- 2 lb. beef, cubed
- 1/2 cup olive oil
- 1 lemon, juice only
- 3 cloves garlic, minced
- 1 onion, sliced
- 1 teaspoon oregano, dried
- 1/4 teaspoon dried thyme,
- 1 teaspoon salt
- 1/4 teaspoon black pepper
- 1 tablespoon parsley, chopped
- 1 cup Worcestershire sauce

Directions

1. Toss beef with the rest of the kebab ingredients in a bowl.
2. Cover the beef and marinate it for 30 minutes.
3. Thread the beef and veggies on the skewers alternately.
4. Place these beef skewers in the Air fry basket. Brush the skewers with the Worcestershire sauce. Press "Power Button" of Air Fry Oven and turn the dial to select the "Air fryer" mode.
5. Press the Time button and again turn the dial to set the cooking time to 20 minutes. Now push the Temp button and rotate the dial to set the temperature at 370 degrees F.
6. Once preheated, place the Air fryer basket in the oven and close its lid.
7. Flip the skewers when cooked halfway through then resume cooking.
8. Serve warm.

BEEF KEBOBS WITH CREAM DIP

Total Time: 30 minutes
Serves: 6

Ingredients

- Beef Kebabs
- 2 lbs. beef, diced
- 1 large onion, squares
- Salt

For the Dressing

- 1 tablespoon mayonnaise
- 1 tablespoon olive oil
- 2 tablespoons lemon juice
- 1 teaspoon yellow mustard
- 1/4 teaspoon salt
- 1/8 teaspoon black pepper

Directions

1. Toss beef and onion with salt in a bowl to season them.
2. Thread the beef and onion on the skewers alternately.
3. Place these beef skewers in the Air fry basket.
4. Press "Power Button" of Air Fry Oven and turn the dial to select the "Air fryer" mode. Press the Time button and again turn the dial to set the cooking time to 20 minutes.
5. Now push the Temp button and rotate the dial to set the temperature at 370 degrees F. Once preheated, place the Air fryer basket in the oven and close its lid. Flip the skewers when cooked halfway through then resume cooking.
6. Prepare the cream dip by mixing its ingredients in a bowl.
7. Serve skewers with cream dip.

ASIAN BEEF SKEWERS

Total Time: 25 minutes
Serves: 4

Ingredients

- 3 tablespoons hoisin sauce
- 3 tablespoons sherry
- 1/4 cup soy sauce
- 1 teaspoon barbeque sauce
- 2 green onions, chopped
- 2 cloves garlic, minced
- 1 tablespoon minced fresh ginger root
- 1 1/2 lbs. flank steak, cubed

Directions

1. Toss steak cubes with sherry, all the sauces and other ingredients in a bowl.
2. Marinate the saucy spiced skewers for 30 minutes.
3. Place these beef skewers in the Air fry basket.
4. Press "Power Button" of Air Fry Oven and turn the dial to select the "Air fryer" mode.
5. Press the Time button and again turn the dial to set the cooking time to 15 minutes.
6. Now push the Temp button and rotate the dial to set the temperature at 350 degrees F.
7. Once preheated, place the Air fryer basket in the oven and close its lid.
8. Flip the skewers when cooked halfway through then resume cooking.
9. Serve warm.

KOREAN BBQ SKEWERS

Total Time: 25 minutes

Serves: 4

Ingredients

- 3 oz. lean sirloin steaks, cubed
- 1 small onion, finely diced
- 1/3 cup low sodium soy sauce
- 1/3 cup brown sugar
- 1 tablespoon sesame seeds
- 2 teaspoons sesame oil
- 4 cloves garlic, diced
- 1 tablespoon ginger, grated
- 1 teaspoon sriracha
- 2 tablespoons honey
- salt and pepper

Directions

1. Toss steak cubes with sauces and other ingredients in a bowl.
2. Marinate the saucy spiced skewers for 30 minutes.
3. Place these beef skewers in the Air fry basket.
4. Press "Power Button" of Air Fry Oven and turn the dial to select the "Air fryer" mode.
5. Press the Time button and again turn the dial to set the cooking time to 15 minutes.
6. Now push the Temp button and rotate the dial to set the temperature at 350 degrees F.
7. Once preheated, place the Air fryer basket in the oven and close its lid.
8. Flip the skewers when cooked halfway through then resume cooking.
9. Serve warm.

ROASTED BEEF BRISKET

Total Time: 100minutes
Serves: 12

Ingredients

- 6 lb. beef brisket, boneless

Spice rub:

- 1 cup olive oil
- juice of 1 lemon
- 1 teaspoon thyme
- 5 teaspoon minced garlic
- Salt to taste
- Black pepper to taste
- 1 stick butter, melted
- 1/2 cup olive oil
- 1 oz. soy sauce
- 1 oz. brown sugar
- 1tbs. black pepper

Directions

1. Place the beef brisket in a baking tray. Whisk spice rub ingredients in a bowl
2. Liberally brush the brisket with the spice mixture.
3. Whisk the baste ingredients in a bowl and keep it aside.
4. Press "Power Button" of Air Fry Oven and turn the dial to select the "Air Roast" mode. Press the Time button and again turn the dial to set the cooking time to 1 hr. 30 minutes.
5. Now push the Temp button and rotate the dial to set the temperature at 370 degrees F. Once preheated, place the beef baking tray in the oven and close its lid. Serve warm.

PORK SKEWERS WITH GARDEN SALAD

Total Time: 30 minutes

Serves: 4

Ingredients

- 1 ¼ lb. boneless pork, diced
- 2 teaspoons balsamic vinegar
- 2 tablespoons olive oil
- 1 garlic clove, crushed

For the salad

- 4 large tomatoes, chopped
- 1 cucumber, chopped
- 1 handful black olives, chopped
- 9 oz. pack feta cheese, crumbled
- 1 bunch of parsley, chopped

Directions

1. Whisk balsamic vinegar with garlic and olive oil in a bowl.
2. Toss in pork cubes and mix well to coat. Marinate for 30 minutes.
3. Alternatively, thread the pork on the skewers.
4. Place these pork skewers in the Air fry basket.
5. Press "Power Button" of Air Fry Oven and turn the dial to select the "Air fryer" mode. Press the Time button and again turn the dial to set the cooking time to 20 minutes.
6. Now push the Temp button and rotate the dial to set the temperature at 360 degrees F. Once preheated, place the Air fryer basket in the oven and close its lid. Flip the skewers when cooked halfway through then resume cooking.
7. Meanwhile, whisk all the salad ingredients in a salad bowl.
8. Serve the skewers with prepared salad.

WINE SOAKED PORK KEBOBS

Total Time: 30 minutes
Serves: 6

Ingredients

- 2 ¼ lbs. pork shoulder, diced
- 1/3 cup avocado oil
- ½ cup red wine
- 2 teaspoon dried oregano
- zest and juice 2 limes
- 2 garlic cloves, crushed

Directions

1. Whisk avocado oil, red wine, oregano, lime juice, zest, and garlic in a suitable bowl.
2. Toss in pork cubes and mix well to coat. Marinate for 30 minutes.
3. Alternatively, thread the pork, onion, and bread on the skewers.
4. Place these pork skewers in the Air fry basket.
5. Press "Power Button" of Air Fry Oven and turn the dial to select the "Air fryer" mode.
6. Press the Time button and again turn the dial to set the cooking time to 20 minutes.
7. Now push the Temp button and rotate the dial to set the temperature at 370 degrees F.
8. Once preheated, place the Air fryer basket in the oven and close its lid.
9. Flip the skewers when cooked halfway through then resume cooking.
10. Serve warm.

PORK SAUSAGES

Total Time: 26 minutes

Serves: 6

Ingredients

- 1 lb. pork mince
- 2 oz. feta cheese
- 1 large red onion, chopped
- ¼ cup parsley, chopped
- ¼ cup mint, chopped
- 1 tablespoon olive oil
- juice 1 lemon

Directions

1. Whisk pork mince with onion, feta, and everything in a bowl.
2. Make 12 sausages out of this mixture then thread them on the skewers.
3. Place these pork skewers in the Air fry basket.
4. Press "Power Button" of Air Fry Oven and turn the dial to select the "Bake" mode.
5. Press the Time button and again turn the dial to set the cooking time to 16 minutes.
6. Now push the Temp button and rotate the dial to set the temperature at 370 degrees F.
7. Once preheated, place the Air fryer basket in the oven and close its lid.
8. Flip the skewers when cooked halfway through then resume cooking.
9. Serve warm.

PEST PORK KEBOBS

Total Time: 30 minutes
Serves: 4

Ingredients

- 9 ½ oz. couscous, boiled
- 2 tablespoon pesto paste
- 2/3 lb. pork steak, diced
- 2 red peppers, cut into chunks
- 2 red onions, cut into chunks
- 1 tablespoon olive oil

Directions

1. Toss in pork cubes with pesto and oil, then mix well to coat. Marinate for 30 minutes.
2. Alternatively, thread the pork, onion, and peppers on the skewers.
3. Place these pork skewers in the Air fry basket.
4. Press "Power Button" of Air Fry Oven and turn the dial to select the "Air fryer" mode.
5. Press the Time button and again turn the dial to set the cooking time to 20 minutes.
6. Now push the Temp button and rotate the dial to set the temperature at 370 degrees F.
7. Once preheated, place the Air fryer basket in the oven and close its lid.
8. Flip the skewers when cooked halfway through then resume cooking.
9. Serve warm with couscous.

PORK SAUSAGE WITH YOGURT DIP

Total Time: 20 minutes
Serves: 8

Ingredients

- 2 tablespoon cumin seed
- 2 tablespoon coriander seed
- 2 tablespoon fennel seed
- 1 tablespoon paprika
- 4 garlic cloves, minced
- ½ teaspoon ground cinnamon
- 1 ½ lb. lean minced pork

For the yogurt

- 3 zucchinis, grated
- 2 teaspoon cumin seed, toasted
- 9 oz. Greek yogurt
- small handful chopped the coriander
- a small handful of chopped mint

Directions

1. Blend all the spices and seeds with garlic and cinnamon in a blender.
2. Add this spice paste to the minced pork then mix well.
3. Make 8 sausages and thread each on the skewers.
4. Place these pork skewers in the Air fry basket.
5. Press "Power Button" of Air Fry Oven and turn the dial to select the "Air fryer" mode. Press the Time button and again turn the dial to set the cooking time to 10 minutes. Now push the Temp button and rotate the dial to set the temperature at 370 degrees F.
6. Once preheated, place the Air fryer basket in the oven and close its lid.
7. Flip the skewers when cooked halfway through then resume cooking.
8. Prepare the yogurt ingredients in a bowl.
9. Serve skewers with the yogurt mixture.

SNACKS & APPETIZERS

RISOTTO BITES

Total Time: 25 minutes

Serves: 4

Ingredients

- 1½ cups cooked risotto
- 3 tablespoons Parmesan cheese, grated
- ½ egg, beaten
- 1½ oz. mozzarella cheese, cubed
- 1/3 cup breadcrumbs

Directions

1. In a bowl, add the risotto, Parmesan and egg and mix until well combined.
2. Make 20 equal-sized balls from the mixture.
3. Insert a mozzarella cube in the center of each ball.
4. With your fingers smooth the risotto mixture to cover the ball.
5. In a shallow dish, place the breadcrumbs.
6. Coat the balls with the breadcrumbs evenly.
7. Press "Power Button" of Air Fry Oven and turn the dial to select the "Air Fry" mode.
8. Press the Time button and again turn the dial to set the cooking time to 10 minutes.
9. Now push the Temp button and rotate the dial to set the temperature at 390 degrees F.
10. Press "Start/Pause" button to start.
11. When the unit beeps to show that it is preheated, open the lid.
12. Arrange the balls in "Air Fry Basket" and insert in the oven.
13. Serve warm.

RICE FLOUR BITES

Total Time: 27 minutes

Serves: 4

Ingredients

- 6 tablespoons milk
- ½ teaspoon vegetable oil
- ¾ cup rice flour
- 1 oz. Parmesan cheese, shredded

Directions

1. In a bowl, add milk, flour, oil and cheese and mix until a smooth dough forms.
2. Make small equal-sized balls from the dough.
3. Press "Power Button" of Air Fry Oven and turn the dial to select the "Air Fry" mode.
4. Press the Time button and again turn the dial to set the cooking time to 12 minutes.
5. Now push the Temp button and rotate the dial to set the temperature at 300 degrees F.
6. Press "Start/Pause" button to start.
7. When the unit beeps to show that it is preheated, open the lid.
8. Arrange the balls in "Air Fry Basket" and insert in the oven.
9. Serve warm.

POTATO CROQUETTES

Total Time: 23 minutes
Serves: 4

Ingredients

- 2 medium Russet potatoes, peeled and cubed
- 2 tablespoons all-purpose flour
- ½ cup Parmesan cheese, grated
- 1 egg yolk
- 2 tablespoons chives, minced
- Pinch of ground nutmeg
- Salt and freshly ground black pepper, as needed
- 2 eggs
- ½ cup breadcrumbs
- 2 tablespoons vegetable oil

Directions

1. In a pan of a boiling water, add the potatoes and cook for about 15 minutes. Drain the potatoes well and transfer into a large bowl.
2. With a potato masher, mash the potatoes and set aside to cool completely.
3. In the bowl of mashed potatoes, add the flour, Parmesan cheese, egg yolk, chives, nutmeg, salt, and black pepper and mix until well combined.
4. Make small equal-sized balls from the mixture.
5. Now, roll each ball into a cylinder shape.
6. In a shallow dish, crack the eggs and beat well.
7. In another dish, mix together the breadcrumbs, and oil. Dip the croquettes in egg mixture and then coat with the breadcrumbs mixture. Press "Power Button" of Air Fry Oven and turn the dial to select the "Air Fry" mode.
8. Press the Time button and again turn the dial to set the cooking time to 8 minutes. Now push the Temp button and rotate the dial to set the temperature at 390 degrees F.
9. Press "Start/Pause" button to start. When the unit beeps to show that it is preheated, open the lid. Arrange the croquettes in "Air Fry Basket" and insert in the oven. Serve warm.

SALMON CROQUETTES

Total Time: 22 minutes
Serves: 8

Ingredients

- ½ of large can red salmon, drained
- 1 egg, lightly beaten
- 1 tablespoon fresh parsley, chopped
- Salt and freshly ground black pepper, as needed
- 3 tablespoons vegetable oil
- ½ cup breadcrumbs

Directions

1. In a bowl, add the salmon and with a fork, mash it completely.
2. Add the eggs, parsley, salt, and black pepper and mix until well combined.
3. Make 8 equal-sized croquettes from the mixture.
4. In a shallow dish, mix together the oil, and breadcrumbs.
5. Coat the croquettes with the breadcrumb mixture.
6. Press "Power Button" of Air Fry Oven and turn the dial to select the "Air Fry" mode.
7. Press the Time button and again turn the dial to set the cooking time to 7 minutes.
8. Now push the Temp button and rotate the dial to set the temperature at 390 degrees F.
9. Press "Start/Pause" button to start.
10. When the unit beeps to show that it is preheated, open the lid.
11. Arrange the croquettes in "Air Fry Basket" and insert in the oven.
12. Serve warm.

BACON CROQUETTES

Total Time: 23 minutes
Serves: 8

Ingredients

- 1 pound sharp cheddar cheese block
- 1 pound thin bacon slices
- 1 cup all-purpose flour
- 3 eggs
- 1 cup breadcrumbs
- Salt, as required
- ¼ cup olive oil

Directions

1. Cut the cheese block into 1-inch rectangular pieces.
2. Wrap 2 bacon slices around 1 piece of cheddar cheese, covering completely.
3. Repeat with the remaining bacon and cheese pieces.
4. Arrange the croquettes in a baking dish and freeze for about 5 minutes.
5. In a shallow dish, place the flour.
6. In a second dish, crack the eggs and beat well.
7. In a third dish, mix together the breadcrumbs, salt, and oil.
8. Coat the croquettes with flour, then dip into beaten eggs and finally, coat with the breadcrumbs mixture.
9. Press "Power Button" of Air Fry Oven and turn the dial to select the "Air Fry" mode. Press the Time button and again turn the dial to set the cooking time to 8 minutes.
10. Now push the Temp button and rotate the dial to set the temperature at 390 degrees F. Press "Start/Pause" button to start.
11. When the unit beeps to show that it is preheated, open the lid.
12. Arrange the croquettes in "Air Fry Basket" and insert in the oven.
13. Serve warm.

CHICKEN NUGGETS

Total Time: 25 minutes
Serves: 6

Ingredients
- 2 large chicken breasts, cut into 1-inch cubes
- 1 cup breadcrumbs
- 1/3 tablespoon Parmesan cheese, shredded
- 1 teaspoon onion powder
- ¼ teaspoon smoked paprika
- Salt and ground black pepper, as required

Directions
1. In a large resealable bag, add all the ingredients.
2. Seal the bag and shake well to coat completely.
3. Press "Power Button" of Air Fry Oven and turn the dial to select the "Air Fry" mode.
4. Press the Time button and again turn the dial to set the cooking time to 10 minutes.
5. Now push the Temp button and rotate the dial to set the temperature at 400 degrees F.
6. Press "Start/Pause" button to start.
7. When the unit beeps to show that it is preheated, open the lid.
8. Arrange the nuggets in "Air Fry Basket" and insert in the oven.
9. Serve warm.

CHICKEN & VEGGIE NUGGETS

Total Time: 30 minutes

Serves: 4

Ingredients

- ½ of zucchini, roughly chopped
- ½ of carrot, roughly chopped
- 14 oz. chicken breast, cut into chunks
- ½ tablespoon mustard powder
- 1 tablespoon garlic powder
- 1 tablespoon onion powder
- Salt and freshly ground black pepper, as needed
- 1 cup all-purpose flour
- 2 tablespoons milk
- 1 egg
- 1 cup panko breadcrumbs

Directions

1. In a food processor, add the zucchini, and carrot and pulse until finely chopped. Add the chicken, mustard powder, garlic powder, onion powder, salt, and black pepper and pulse until well combined.
2. In a shallow dish, place the flour.
3. In a second dish, mix together the milk, and egg.
4. In a third dish, put the breadcrumbs.
5. Coat the nuggets with flour, then dip into egg mixture and finally, coat with the breadcrumbs. Press "Power Button" of Air Fry Oven and turn the dial to select the "Air Fry" mode. Press the Time button and again turn the dial to set the cooking time to 10 minutes.
6. Now push the Temp button and rotate the dial to set the temperature at 390 degrees F. Press "Start/Pause" button to start.
7. When the unit beeps to show that it is preheated, open the lid.
8. Arrange the nuggets in "Air Fry Basket" and insert in the oven.
9. Serve warm.

COD NUGGETS

Total Time: 23 minutes

Serves: 5

Ingredients

- 1 cup all-purpose flour
- 2 eggs
- ¾ cup breadcrumbs
- Pinch of salt
- 2 tablespoons olive oil
- 1 lb. cod, cut into 1x2½-inch strips

Directions

1. In a shallow dish, place the flour.
2. Crack the eggs in a second dish and beat well.
3. In a third dish, mix together the breadcrumbs, salt, and oil.
4. Coat the nuggets with flour, then dip into beaten eggs and finally, coat with the breadcrumbs.
5. Press "Power Button" of Air Fry Oven and turn the dial to select the "Air Fry" mode.
6. Press the Time button and again turn the dial to set the cooking time to 8 minutes.
7. Now push the Temp button and rotate the dial to set the temperature at 390 degrees F.
8. Press "Start/Pause" button to start.
9. When the unit beeps to show that it is preheated, open the lid.
10. Arrange the nuggets in "Air Fry Basket" and insert in the oven.
11. Serve warm.

BBQ CHICKEN WINGS

Total Time: 34 minutes
Serves: 4

Ingredients

- 2 lbs. chicken wings
- 1 teaspoon olive oil
- 1 teaspoon smoked paprika
- 1 teaspoon garlic powder
- Salt and ground black pepper, as required
- ¼ cup BBQ sauce

Directions

1. In a large bowl combine chicken wings, smoked paprika, garlic powder, oil, salt, and pepper and mix well.
2. Press "Power Button" of Air Fry Oven and turn the dial to select the "Air Fry" mode.
3. Press the Time button and again turn the dial to set the cooking time to 19 minutes.
4. Now push the Temp button and rotate the dial to set the temperature at 360 degrees F.
5. Press "Start/Pause" button to start.
6. When the unit beeps to show that it is preheated, open the lid.
7. Arrange the chicken wings in "Air Fry Basket" and insert in the oven.
8. After 12 minutes of cooking, flip the wings and coat with barbecue sauce evenly.
9. Serve immediately.

BUFFALO CHICKEN WINGS

Total Time: 31 minutes

Serves: 5

Ingredients

- 2 lbs. frozen chicken wings, drums and flats separated
- 2 tablespoons olive oil
- 2 tablespoons Buffalo sauce
- ½ teaspoon red pepper flakes, crushed
- Salt, as required

Directions

1. Coat the chicken wings with oi evenly.
2. Press "Power Button" of Air Fry Oven and turn the dial to select the "Air Fry" mode.
3. Press the Time button and again turn the dial to set the cooking time to 16 minutes.
4. Now push the Temp button and rotate the dial to set the temperature at 390 degrees F.
5. Press "Start/Pause" button to start.
6. When the unit beeps to show that it is preheated, open the lid.
7. Arrange the chicken wings in "Air Fry Basket" and insert in the oven.
8. After 12 minutes of cooking, flip the wings and coat with barbecue sauce evenly.
9. After 7 minutes, flip the wings.
10. Meanwhile, in a large bowl, add Buffalo sauce, red pepper flakes and salt and mix well.
11. Transfer the wings into the bowl of Buffalo sauce and toss to coat well.
12. Serve immediately.

CRISPY PRAWNS

Total Time: 23 minutes

Serves: 4

Ingredients

- 1 egg
- ½ pound nacho chips, crushed
- 12 prawns, peeled and deveined

Directions

1. In a shallow dish, beat the egg.
2. In another shallow dish, place the crushed nacho chips.
3. Coat the prawn into egg and then roll into nacho chips.
4. Press "Power Button" of Air Fry Oven and turn the dial to select the "Air Fry" mode.
5. Press the Time button and again turn the dial to set the cooking time to 8 minutes.
6. Now push the Temp button and rotate the dial to set the temperature at 355 degrees F.
7. Press "Start/Pause" button to start.
8. When the unit beeps to show that it is preheated, open the lid.
9. Arrange the prawns in "Air Fry Basket" and insert in the oven.
10. Serve immediately.

BREADED SHRIMP

Total Time: 22 minutes

Serves: 4

Ingredients

- 8 large shrimp, peeled and deveined
- Salt and ground black pepper, as required
- 8 ounces coconut milk
- ½ cup panko breadcrumbs
- ½ teaspoon cayenne pepper

Directions

1. In a shallow dish, mix together salt, black pepper and coconut milk.
2. In another shallow dish, mix together breadcrumbs, cayenne pepper, salt and black pepper.
3. Dip the shrimp in coconut milk mixture and then roll into breadcrumbs mixture.
4. Press "Power Button" of Air Fry Oven and turn the dial to select the "Air Fry" mode.
5. Press the Time button and again turn the dial to set the cooking time to 12 minutes.
6. Now push the Temp button and rotate the dial to set the temperature at 350 degrees F.
7. Press "Start/Pause" button to start.
8. When the unit beeps to show that it is preheated, open the lid.
9. Arrange the shrimp in "Air Fry Basket" and insert in the oven.
10. Serve immediately.

BACON WRAPPED SHRIMP

Total Time: 22 minutes

Serves: 6

Ingredients

- 1 lb. bacon, sliced thinly
- 1 lb. shrimp, peeled and deveined

Directions

1. Wrap one slice of bacon around each shrimp completely.
2. Arrange the shrimp in a baking dish and refrigerate for about 20 minutes.
3. Press "Power Button" of Air Fry Oven and turn the dial to select the "Air Fry" mode.
4. Press the Time button and again turn the dial to set the cooking time to 6 minutes.
5. Now push the Temp button and rotate the dial to set the temperature at 390 degrees F.
6. Press "Start/Pause" button to start.
7. When the unit beeps to show that it is preheated, open the lid.
8. Arrange the shrimp in "Air Fry Basket" and insert in the oven.
9. Serve immediately.

FETA TATER TOTS

Total Time: 40 minutes
Serves: 6

Ingredients

- 2 lbs. frozen tater tots
- ½ cup feta cheese, crumbled
- ½ cup tomato, chopped
- ¼ cup black olives, pitted and sliced
- ¼ cup red onion, chopped

Directions

1. Press "Power Button" of Air Fry Oven and turn the dial to select the "Air Fry" mode.
2. Press the Time button and again turn the dial to set the cooking time to 25 minutes.
3. Now push the Temp button and rotate the dial to set the temperature at 450 degrees F.
4. Press "Start/Pause" button to start.
5. When the unit beeps to show that it is preheated, open the lid.
6. Arrange the tater tots in "Air Fry Basket" and insert in the oven.
7. After 15 minutes of cooking, press "Start/Pause" button to pause the unit
8. Remove basket from oven and transfer tots into a large bowl.
9. Add the feta cheese, tomatoes, olives and onion and toss to coat well.
10. Now, place the mixture into "Sheet Pan" and insert in the oven.
11. Press "Start/Pause" button to resume cooking.
12. Serve warm.

BUTTERMILK BISCUITS

Total Time: 23 minutes
Serves: 8

Ingredients

- ½ cup cake flour
- 1¼ cups all-purpose flour
- ¼ teaspoon baking soda
- ½ teaspoon baking powder
- 1 teaspoon granulated sugar
- Salt, to taste
- ¼ cup cold unsalted butter, cut into cubes
- ¾ cup buttermilk
- 2 tablespoons butter, melted

Directions

1. In a large bowl, sift together flours, baking soda, baking powder, sugar and salt. With a pastry cutter, cut cold butter and mix until a coarse crumb forms. Slowly, add buttermilk and mix until a smooth dough forms.
2. Place the dough onto a floured surface and with your hands, press it into ½ inch thickness.
3. With a 1¾-inch round cookie cutter, cut the biscuits.
4. Arrange the biscuits into a baking pan in a single layer and coat with the butter. Press "Power Button" of Air Fry Oven and turn the dial to select the "Air Fry" mode. Press the Time button and again turn the dial to set the cooking time to 8 minutes.
5. Now push the Temp button and rotate the dial to set the temperature at 400 degrees F. Press "Start/Pause" button to start.
6. When the unit beeps to show that it is preheated, open the lid. Arrange pan over the "Wire Rack" and insert in the oven. Place the baking pan onto a wire rack for about 5 minutes. Carefully, invert the biscuits onto the wire rack to cool completely before serving.

DESSERT RECIPES

SESAME BANANA DESSERT

Total Time: 15 minutes

Serves: 5

Ingredients
- 1 ½ cups flour
- 5 bananas, sliced
- 1 tsp salt
- 3 tbsp sesame seeds
- 1 cup water
- 2 eggs, beaten
- 1 tsp baking powder
- ½ tbsp sugar

Directions
Preheat Cuisinart on Bake function to 340 F. In a bowl, mix salt, sesame seeds, flour, baking powder, eggs, sugar, and water. Coat sliced bananas with the flour mixture. Place the prepared slices in the Air Fryer basket and fit in the baking tray; cook for 8-10 minutes. Serve chilled.

TRIPLE BERRY LEMON CRUMBLE

Total Time: 30 minutes
Serves: 6

Ingredients

- 12 oz fresh strawberries
- 7 oz fresh raspberries
- 5 oz fresh blueberries
- 5 tbsp cold butter
- 2 tbsp lemon juice
- 1 cup flour
- ½ cup sugar
- 1 tbsp water
- A pinch of salt

Directions

1. Gently mash the berries, but make sure there are chunks left. Mix with the lemon juice and 2 tbsp of the sugar. Place the berry mixture at the bottom of a prepared round cake.

2. Combine the flour with the salt and sugar in a bowl. Add the water and rub the butter with your fingers until the mixture becomes crumbled. Pour the batter over the berries. Cook in your Cuisinart at 390 F for 20 minutes on Bake function. Serve chilled.

HONEY HAZELNUT APPLES

Total Time: 13 minutes
Serves: 4

Ingredients
- 4 apples
- 1 oz butter
- 2 oz breadcrumbs
- Zest of 1 orange
- 2 tbsp chopped hazelnuts
- 2 oz mixed seeds
- 1 tsp cinnamon
- 2 tbsp honey

Directions
Preheat Cuisinart on Bake function to 350 F. Core the apples. Make sure to also score their skin to prevent from splitting. Combine the remaining ingredients in a bowl; stuff the apples with the mixture and cook for 10 minutes. Serve topped with chopped hazelnuts.

FRENCH APPLE CAKE

Total Time: 25 minutes

Serves: 9

Ingredients

- 2 ¾ oz flour
- 5 tbsp sugar
- 1 ¼ oz butter
- 3 tbsp cinnamon
- 2 whole apple, sliced

Directions

1. Preheat Cuisinart on Bake function to 360 F. In a bowl, mix 3 tbsp sugar, butter, and flour and form a pastry dough. Roll out the pastry on a floured surface and transfer it to the fryer's baking dish. Arrange the apple slices atop.

2. Cover the apples with sugar and cinnamon and cook for 20 minutes. Sprinkle with powdered sugar and mint and serve.

CLASSIC PECAN PIE

Total Time: 1 hr 10 minutes

Serves: 3-4

Ingredients

- ¾ cup maple syrup
- 2 eggs
- ½ tsp salt
- ¼ tsp nutmeg
- ½ tsp cinnamon
- 2 tbsp almond butter
- 2 tbsp brown sugar
- ½ cup chopped pecans
- 1 tbsp butter, melted
- 1 8-inch pie dough
- ¾ tsp vanilla extract

Directions

1. Preheat Cuisinart on Toast function to 350 F. Coat the pecans with the melted butter. Place the pecans in a baking tray and toast them for 5 minutes. Place the pie crust into the baking pan, and scatter the pecans over.

2. Whisk together all remaining ingredients in a bowl. Pour the maple mixture over the pecans. Set Cuisinart to 320 F and cook the pie for 25 minutes on Bake function.

AUTHENTIC RAISIN APPLE TREAT

Total Time: 15 minutes
Serves: 4

Ingredients
- 4 apples, cored
- 1 ½ oz almonds
- ¾ oz raisins
- 2 tbsp sugar

Directions
Preheat Cuisinart on Bake function to 360 F. In a bowl, mix sugar, almonds, and raisins. Blend the mixture using a hand mixer. Fill cored apples with the almond mixture. Place the apples in a baking tray and cook for 10 minutes. Serve with a sprinkle of powdered sugar.

CRUMBLE WITH BLACKBERRIES & APRICOTS

Total Time: 30 minutes

Serves: 4

Ingredients

- 2 ½ cups fresh apricots, cubed
- 1 cup fresh blackberries
- ½ cup sugar
- 2 tbsp lemon Juice
- 1 cup flour
- 5 tbsp butter

Directions

Preheat Cuisinart on Bake function to 390 F. Add apricots to a bowl and mix with lemon juice, 2 tbsp sugar, and blackberries. Spread the mixture onto the greased Air Fryer baking pan. In another bowl, mix flour and remaining sugar. Add 1 tbsp of cold water and butter and keep mixing until you have a crumbly mixture; top with crumb mixture. Cook for 20 minutes.

CPSIA information can be obtained
at www.ICGtesting.com
Printed in the USA
BVHW012219240820
586989BV00041B/228